An Essenti(to Health Insurance for Companies

A KEY TOOL TO ASSIST COMPANY
LEADERS MAKE INFORMED CHOICES TO
BENEFIT THEIR STAFF

Best Wishes **Isaac Feiner**

www.lifepointhealthcare.co.uk

THIS IS A MARKETING COMMUNICATION

Isaac Feiner
isaac@lifepointhealthcare.co.uk

Ordering Information:
Quantity sales. Special discounts are available on quantity purchases by corporations, associations, and others. For details, contact the "Special Sales Department" at the email address above.

An Essential Guide to Health Insurance for Companies/ Isaac Feiner. —1st ed.
ISBN 9781796441185

Contents

INTRODUCTION

This guide is about choosing and buying company health insurance for yourself, your family and staff. It's an important purchase and there's no doubt that if you are better informed and able to dispel any confusion you may have about the terms used and the options on offer, your ultimate decision can be made with greater peace of mind and lead to a happy, smooth sailing outcome for all involved.

The industry abounds with a mass of conflicting information and wading through it can be daunting and time-consuming. This short, user-friendly book is designed to offer knowledge and understanding at your fingertips, making this annual process less of a burden and so freeing you up to for other matters within your business.

My knowledge and expertise have been built up over many years in the industry. I've helped thousands of people, hundreds of companies (large and small), nurtured millions of pounds of premiums and immersed myself in various aspects of the health insurance broking sector.

I take pride in my work as Founder and Director of Lifepoint Healthcare where I am an impartial intermediary for all my new and long-standing clients.

It's this role as well as my position as Executive Committee Member of the Association of Medical Insurers and Intermediaries (AMII), which has given me the firm foundation needed to share with you this overview with knowledge, insight and understanding, and also with clarity and impartiality.

Whether you choose to use this as a handy reference tool or read it cover to cover, I hope it helps.

Why Buy Health Insurance?

If you concur that a key asset within your business is your staff, then investing in their wellbeing is crucial to driving that business forward.

The benefits of Private Medical Insurance can do much to reduce staff absence through sickness, medical appointments with long NHS waiting times and quite simply serve to instil a general feeling of well-being, as well as ensuring staff feel appreciated and looked after. If Mental Health issues are also addressed within the plan, the positive impact this provision can provide, will only serve to enhance and strengthen a modern-day workforce.

Taking things a step further, offering benefits such as these can help you to attract the right staffing talent and retain them, especially when your competitors are not offering this as part of their employee benefits package.

While the corporate landscape still has the uncertainty of Brexit to deal with, the rising momentum to improve employee health provides favourable dynamics for increased spend on healthcare benefits by companies.

LaingBuisson – health intelligence provider
Health Cover UK Market Report Oct 2018

In short, a valued employee is a happy employee which filters down throughout your business and the bottom line value it can reap.

The Next Step to Staff Wellbeing

It's time to consider or review your existing healthcare arrangements.

But not before you've read this book.

It's tempting to go online, fish about, click on companies at the top of search engines and dip into a host of subject-related articles. You may reach a landing page, fill in some details for a quote and click send, often into a void of uncertainty. Messages can flood your inbox and leave you with a web of messages and information to unravel.

There is nothing wrong with a sales team eager to help you, but it's the uncertainty of who and what to trust and the fact that you are given so many different options that can really grate.

Or you may already have a healthcare plan in place but how often is it carefully reviewed in terms of its benefits and value for money? I've heard stories from new company clients wanting a full review of their existing policy. What they had experienced was their employees would go to claim and find their cover was not robust enough, lacked certain benefits or had limited cover. This left a sour taste in their staff's mouths and therefore, also a negative view of their employer, who was only trying to do good by offering it in the first place. More pain.

The impartial knowledge therefore I humbly impart is your next step. Presented in the following pages is an expert, well-founded overview of the various elements in the private health insurance purchasing journey.

May this help you and allow you to make the right healthcare decisions for your company, resulting in happy employees, a thriving business, massive growth, revenues and even bigger profits.

Empowered with this information, I offer you blessings for continued health.

Isaac Feiner
London, 2019

CHAPTER 1

Price, Cover & Underwriting

As price is an important part of the buying process I want to address this first. In this chapter I am going to show you how you should think about and approach the cost of your firm's private medical insurance premium, whether it is your existing policy coming up for renewal or if you are considering the provision of private health insurance for the first time. This should give you more clarity in helping to make your decisions and choices.

As it stands, clients are concerned about the rising costs of healthcare and rightfully so. Year on year, even without claims being made during the policy year, policies can see an average 10 -20% increase. This can be far higher when claims have been made (upwards of even 65-70%), so it is important to know how to structure a plan when taking out a new policy as well as how to deal with the price with regards to your renewal.

I believe that price should not be the absolute focus of a purchase and my experience dealing with professionals is that this is a shared sentiment. The issue of price tends to be a myth because whilst as a buyer you may be shopping at the lowest price, it is value that you truly want. And when value exceeds the price, then suddenly price no longer remains the issue. However, cost does still tend to be one of the biggest concerns for people and companies when dealing with an expensive purchase like private medical insurance, so here goes.

The Make Up of a Health Insurance Policy

The premium cost is affected by the actual benefits chosen in any given plan. The premise being the more comprehensive the level of cover, the higher the cost.

Policies tend to be modular, meaning you begin with a standard baseline of cover and can pick and choose to add additional benefits if you wish to enhance the cover level. This is where the policy can be 'fleshed' out to maximise benefit and is where you might seek the advice of an experienced professional to guide you on the myriad of options.

A competent adviser would know all the options for each provider and how to structure the plan correctly to minimise cost and maximise benefit.

Generalised Breakdown of Benefits

Each policy will have its own nuances of cover based on the following, so it is always crucial to read the actual policy summary when considering a specific insurer and product.

1. **Inpatient and Day patient benefit:**

This relates to hospital charges for overnight stays and day cases. *This tends to be included as a baseline of core cover for*

most plans. The cover may include hospital charges including accommodation and meals, nursing care, drugs and surgical dressings and theatre fees, diagnostic tests, operating-theatre costs, drugs and dressings, radiotherapy, chemotherapy, and surgical appliances at private hospitals and day-patient units and specialist fees for surgeons, anaesthetists and physicians.

2. **Outpatient benefit**:

This covers specialist consultations with approved specialists, diagnostic tests (including CT/PET/MRI Scans, X-rays, Blood tests, ECG's), fees for practitioners, and can include specialist referred physiotherapy, nurses, dieticians, orthoptists and speech therapists.

3. **Cancer Cover:**

This may include the full cancer treatment pathways including, out-patient diagnostic tests and consultations, radiotherapy, chemotherapy and follow-up consultations, biological therapies, hormone and bisphosphonate therapies, cancer surgery and reconstructive surgery, stem cell therapy, end-of-life home nursing.

Given the cancer epidemic I believe this is an important aspect of any private healthcare plan as lifesaving treatment is exceptionally costly and the peace of mind it provides is important. The claims can be incredibly high when treating cancer so full cover is required to ensure the majority of costs are covered. Although most insurers do now follow the trend of offering comprehensive cancer cover, there are some insurers that will have caveats so it is absolutely vital you ask about any caveats on the cancer cover. As an example, cancer caveats can vary from a limitation on how long a particular type of treatment may be given (biological therapies) or exclude certain treatments completely (bone marrow or stem cell transplants in certain situations).

4. Therapies:

This may include fees for physiotherapy, acupuncture, homeopathy or therapist treatment, osteopathy, chiropractic/podiatry, speech and language therapy.

5. Mental Health:

For treatment of an acute mental or psychiatric illness. This may include In-patient and day-patient treatment, outpatient treatment, psychologists, psychiatrists and cognitive behavioural therapists.

The above are the primary benefits available and there are a variety of additional extra benefits available depending on the insurer. These extra benefits can include:

Dental and Optical benefit, Travel Cover, Private GP, Employee Assistance Programs, and extra membership benefits depending on the insurer etc.

The level of cover for some of the above benefits can also be tailored. For example, you can have a limitation on the use of the outpatient benefit - capped at a financial limit per year or a maximum number of visits to a specialist, or you can have the benefit on a fully comprehensive level which includes no annual limits.

Furthermore, depending on which of above benefits chosen and at what level of cover, the plan and pricing can be tailored a step further depending on the following:

- **Level of excess chosen:**

As a general rule the higher the excess chosen, the lower the premium. Excess amounts can range from £100 to £3000 with many variables in between. An excess can be payable per person per year or per claim (insurer dependant). Or can be a co-payment option, where you pay a percentage of the claim capped at an amount predefined at the time of policy set up.

- **Hospital listings:**

Most insurers will have different levels of hospital listings which will affect the premium. The most costly listing may cover all the London Hospitals. If you do not require the inner London hospitals and are happy with the hundreds of other options, then this is important to consider as a method for cost containment. Insurers do have different lists so it is vital to check that the list covers the facilities you would expect your employees to use in case of a medical situation.

- **The method of underwriting in place (the way the policy was set up):**

These are the primary methods of underwriting. As each method poses a different risk to the insurer, the choice of underwriting may also affect the premium. This is certainly the case when choosing MHD (Medical History Disregarded) as the insurer is aware they are more vulnerable to paying claims for pre-existing conditions.

Underwriting Methods

1. Moratorium

Different insurers may have slightly different Moratorium wording. The client will not have to fill in a health questionnaire when applying for cover and the medical underwriting is done at point of the claims.

The insurer excludes any conditions for which you have received medication, advice or treatment or for which you have experienced symptoms, whether the condition has been diagnosed or not in the five years before the start of your cover (pre-existing conditions). Related conditions (those which are medically considered to be associated with a pre-existing condition) will also not be covered. However, if you have not had any such symptoms, treatment, medication or advice for pre-existing conditions or any related conditions for a continuous period of two years after the start date of your policy, the condition will become eligible for cover. This period is known as the Moratorium. Though the two year moratorium is most common, some insurers offer other lengths of moratorium.

2. Continued Moratorium (when moving from an existing Moratorium policy)

The moratorium underwriting term of your current insurer will apply and the start date of the moratorium underwriting does not start again. Please note that the benefits and terms and conditions of your new policy will apply and it is only the dates of underwriting with your current insurer that will be matched. There must be no break in insurance cover since underwriting. A switch declaration will also need to be completed to facilitate the transfer. These are questions and criteria that need to be satisfied and allow the new insurer to assess your eligibility to access this method of underwriting. If the eligibility for transfer is not met, the insurer may refuse to offer cover on this form of underwriting.

3. Full Medical Underwriting (FMU)

A health questionnaire is completed on the application form. After reviewing the employee's completed question-naire, the insurer will let them know at the outset the basis on which they can offer cover, listing any pre-existing conditions they may have that would not be covered on the policy. If necessary, they may ask the member's doctor for further information. It is important that joiners list full and accurate information. It is important to focus on answering the questions accurately and completely to make sure that the policy provides valid cover.

4. CPME: Continued Personal Medical Exclusions (Switch)

Plans include continuous cover for pre-existing conditions and are as shown on your current insurer's medical certificate. Exclusions shown on the current certificate will be continued (subject to the terms and conditions of the policy itself). As clients have had prior medical insurance he/she will be covered on CPME (Switch) terms. If there are any declarations made when answering the switch questions, exclusions may be applied. A copy of the current certificate(s) will be required with the application.

5. **Medical History Disregarded (MHD)**

    This method of underwriting allows for pre-existing conditions to be covered without medical exclusions but is still subject to the terms and conditions of the policy. There is a minimum membership number required to set an MHD scheme up and it usually costs more than the above methods of underwriting.

In addition to the above, policies due for renewal increase in costs due to the following:

- **Medical Inflation increases:**

  This is standard on every policy in the UK. Medical inflation is the rising cost of medical treatment across the board. Medical Inflation runs between 6% - 12%.

- **Age Band Increases:**

  As people age, the risk of ill health increases and therefore so does the likelihood of claims costs to the insurer. Most providers account for this by increasing the premiums of individuals as single year age bands at the renewal each year.

- **Insurance Premium Tax:**

  As from 01.11.2015 Insurance premium tax (IPT), increased from 6% to 9.5%, October 2016 from 9.5% to 10% and a further increase of 2% from the 1st of June 2017. We never quite know how stable this figure will remain. (At the last election, Labour was making promises to increase this to 20% if elected). This extra tax was to assist them with shoring up flood defences.

- **Claims made during the year:**

  Claims performance is taken into account at a group level on company schemes. If claims performance exceeds the insurers' target loss ratio (claims paid against premium paid, net of insurance premium tax) then an additional increase may be applied.

As you can see, private healthcare can be a minefield to the business consumer and when carrying out your research you will be faced with multiple options, benefits, levels of cover, underwriting methods, as well as different insurer stances and you will have to take all this into account and distil it into purchasing a product that suits your needs at the right price.

Ideally the provision of a fully comprehensive plan is usually the preferred option so as to cover more eventualities. However, if you know how to structure a plan correctly, it is possible to reduce costs significantly whilst retaining the important benefits to you and your staff. This ideally is where you want to be.

Remember price is important but primarily you need to consider and ask yourself the following:

What is truly important to you as a firm putting a private healthcare plan in place (what outcome are you trying to achieve by offering this benefit)?

Which options and benefits are important to you and your employees (how much cover do you want your plan to provide to the policy members)?

What experience do you want the product to achieve for you and your employees (is it employee retention, overall peace of mind, attracting the best talent to your business)?

Each business will have their own focus about what and why they want to put in place a suitable private healthcare package and it is my job as a specialist to help you find the right cover with the right product at the right price with the right company.

All the options available will influence the level of investment required and you will have to make a decision based on this information.

CHAPTER 2

Myth: Insurance Companies Don't Pay Claims

Let's address the elephant in the room no one wants to talk about.

There is this fear out there that if you take out a company health insurance policy, you are going to pay all these premiums, often for several years and then in a time of crisis find that the insurers won't pay the claim.

I validate this fear and I would like to address this, as regardless as to the actual veracity of the truth of this fear, the fear itself does exist. Certainly, when I talk to people considering taking out private healthcare, either consumers or businesses, this does come up as an objection. In the words of one recent client conversation, "the questionable risk for me buying insurance is will they pay out in the event of a claim, even though I have paid premiums all this time and the claim is legitimate?"

This fear is compounded by stories in the media and perhaps your personal experiences surrounding the use of other insurance products.

Whilst I do acknowledge that there have been occasions in the insurance world when this has happened, I can confirm, based on my experience (being witness to hundreds of claims) that the insurers have very strict guidelines and work hard to ensure claims are assessed fairly to ensure a favorable outcome for the policyholder. I tend to find that the bulk of the misunderstandings occur where there is miscommunication about the claims process, what is covered and eligibility of claims.

Therefore, it is always important for the policyholders to understand the claims process and the terms of their cover to maximise the chances of a claim.

This is also very much the responsibility of the intermediary to explain the nuances of the policy clearly. Whether through clear, jargon free, easy to understand written advice, a presentation, or the dissemination of the insurer key facts, policy documents and more recently, for consumer policies only, the mandatory Insurance Product Information Document that concisely breaks down the policy benefits, what is insured and what is not, including any significant exclusions the client should be aware of.

In my opinion, the general recommended process is that the broker clearly takes the time to break down the benefits of the recommended option and also make a comparison table where necessary. This is the first step for a client actually seeing what the policy and its relevant components are offering.

In my firm, each client receives this type of guidance and we regularly take the time, at length to explain each part of the cover in simple terms, answering questions along the way so as to ensure the client is receiving the correct information and is guided accurately into the purchase.

I tell my specialist team it is crucial to remember that most people are not immersed in the detail like we as specialists are. Indeed, that is precisely why they are coming to us, instead of attempting the purchase of a complex insurance product themselves.

It is also the responsibility of the company/employer/policyholders to try take the time to understand things on their own accord, to understand what they have purchased or what has been purchased on their behalf.

We always advise that before throwing the documents in a drawer, to take the time to read through it and to address any queries or questions the client may have.

Furthermore, the way you can avoid having the above problems and ensuring peace of mind, is by working with a reputable intermediary, who has relationships with the insurance companies.

As a consumer of the product, you may only deal with one, two or three insurers in a lifetime, however I have relationships with the bulk of the insurers so am in a better position to guide appropriately. It is hard for you, the consumer to know the difference. So, it just makes sense for you to take guidance. The same way you would take guidance from professionals on a myriad of other things.

We work with most of the insurance providers and have a large choice of products to choose from on a regular basis. I currently have many clients with the various insurers and we manage a large portfolio so I get to see how the insurers behave and how they treat my customers in all respects. This frontline knowledge guides me when advising clients.

If a company doesn't treat my customers well, I tend to avoid placing business with them. I only want my clients to have a pleasant experience and to be well looked after in the event of an acute medical situation. From a business standpoint, I want loyal, happy, satisfied, cared for clients who stay with us for many years and refer their colleagues at other companies, as well as friends and family.

I would also point out, to maximise the chance of claims being paid, that disclosure of any known issues in the fact-finding pre-sales process is important. These are called Material Facts/Circumstances. It is the adviser's responsibility to draw the customer's attention to the Terms of Business Document and explain the importance of disclosing material circumstances and the potential consequences of non-disclosure.

An example of a material fact is something that the Group Secretary knows about the health of the employees but doesn't disclose to the insurer when asked. Examples are recent and ongoing cancer, heart and psychiatric illness. The impact of non-disclosure can be disastrous and potentially lead to non-payment of claims. So, it is always advisable for the person responsible for setting up the company scheme to disclose facts correctly.

CHAPTER 3

Ensuring Suitability of Cover, Staying Off the NHS Waiting Lists & Getting Access to Doctors & Hospitals

Ok, so you have decided that you want to put some suitable cover in place to protect your employees and possibly their families. Or perhaps you might be reading this and already have a policy in place.

In both cases, as a new or existing policyholder, you want to ask yourself, does the cover in place suit the firm's needs and does it do the job of protecting the workforce adequately, giving the employees peace of mind and a suitable safety net to fall back on in the event of an acute medical necessity?

Getting the right coverage in place is more complicated than you think and is certainly not as simple as say buying a new phone contract. It takes thought and awareness of the details.

Here is some guidance on the kinds of things you want to be looking out for.

Avoiding the NHS Waiting Lists

By definition health insurance in the UK is designed for the treatment of acute medical situations and to get you back to better as soon as possible. It is designed to ensure that the policyholder can be seen quickly, bypass the NHS waiting periods and be seen by a medical practitioner (if the specific insurer criteria are met for which consultant you can see. If the criteria are not met you may not see the actual consultant of your choice), at a time and location of your choosing.

*As it stands, according to researched industry publications and data procured under a Freedom of Information request by the Express, the number of patients who die while on NHS waiting lists each year has surged by 10,000 from five years ago. 67 of the 135 trusts asked for information responded and across all of them, 18,876 people had died while on waiting lists five years ago, but this number has now increased to 29,553 this year (2018). And this statistic has come from only half of England's hospital trusts so the actual figure may well be higher.

*Original source Health Insurance Daily 11/09/18.

The above is crucial, so when choosing the options of a plan, make sure you take into account the various hospitals' listings and availability of specialists with the particular insurer you may be thinking of joining.

Many of my London based clients request that the full comprehensive hospital listing be included in the plan because the inner London facilities are where they would wish to be treated; this higher level of listing increases the premium accordingly to reflect the cost of these said hospitals.

However, clients based outside London, or anywhere else in the UK, may not see the inner London listing as an imperative part of their cover, and provided that the hospital listing they choose has provision to care for them at suitable facilities in their location (of which there are usually many to choose from), they may tend to opt for this listing instead. This most likely will also reduce the cost of the premium.

These insurer hospital lists are easily accessible online and should be sent through to the client by the adviser as part of the advice process. A health insurance specialist will also be able to guide you as to the nuances of the different hospital lists and answer any specific questions that may come up when making a decision about which options to go for.

Protecting Yourself and Your Employees from Cancer

Whilst most policies in the market do place huge emphasis on providing a very robust, comprehensive level of cover for the critical conditions, like heart and cancer related illnesses, care should once again be taken to ensure there are no exclusions or caveats.

If there are any, these should be highlighted and discussed. There is nothing more distressing than finding out a crucial element of cover for a major illness is not available on the policy in time of need and that it did not form part of the presales conversation.

In most cases, my clients want comprehensive cancer cover (having unfortunately seen countless cancer cases including my own mother's three-month terminal battle with liver cancer at age 49) this is an area of cover that ideally should not be compromised or ignored.

Caveats to look out for are any time limits on certain treatments e.g. biological therapies (cancer related), any limitations on experimental treatments, targeted/biological therapies (advanced therapeutics) or bone marrow or stem cell transplants, palliative care, treatment or care for cancer which is described by your oncologist as end of life care (sometimes described as terminal), or even an initial waiting period from the start date for any form of cancer treatment.

Where my company has made a recommendation for a more limited cancer product, this has been highlighted in bright yellow in the report so as to ensure this was brought to the client's attention and care taken to discuss the exclusions and caveats in depth. Our duty of care demands this at the very least.

Getting Access to Doctors

It is also important to assess the listings of specialists and consultants who work with the insurer. Some providers make this very easy by providing an online search function, others can be asked to confirm whether they work with any particular specialists, if necessary. This is also very important if you are currently covered with an insurer and are aware of any ongoing treatment at a particular hospital with a specific doctor. It is worthwhile checking the employee or policy member can continue treatment uninterrupted.

Other major areas of concern should be the heart coverage. Like the cancer treatment, insurers tend to place a very strong level of emphasis of cover and care in this area but it is also prudent to understand the full picture before moving forward with a plan.

It is also exceptionally important to be given guidance on the way the policy works - how easy the insurer makes the claims process i.e. how easy and quickly can the claimant have a claim assessed, authorised, the issues treated and be back to better in as quick amount of time as possible. Ultimately people want an easy journey and to have issues resolved with minimum of fuss. In this case the old adage rings true "whilst you are buying the product you are truly buying the claim".

Covering Common, Everyday Health Issues

Finally, it is also important, to ensure that the smaller everyday healthcare issues can be covered as well. Things like musculoskeletal claims, physiotherapy, dental treatment, optical claims and smaller medical issues that you may normally pay the provider of the treatment cash directly. These tend to be called cash plan benefits and can be either included onto a main plan or alongside, as a separate cash plan bolt-on to the main comprehensive healthcare product.

Additionally, having a cash plan alongside the main health insurance policy can allow you to minimise the use of the private medical insurance plan for the smaller everyday issues and thereby prevent these claims from affecting the premium increases at the annual renewal. Yet another way to ensure that premiums remain as cost effective as possible.

It is difficult for you to know all the ins and outs of all the policies, which is why it is ever important that you have a trusting relationship with the adviser. You need to be able to trust the advice is on point and that the product can ultimately deliver the benefits and provide a suitable solution to solve the problem within a quick timeframe.

All these points above are why we place such emphasis on carrying out a suitable fact-finding process. The fact find is designed to allow us to 'know' you as a client, to understand your needs, problems and to extract any other information that can impact our advice to you.

This means that the solution we put together, suits your needs accurately, so that when a medical issue does arise and your workforce need treatment, care or advice, the policy will prove its worth and benefit you, your employees and company accordingly.

CHAPTER 4

Employee Absenteeism: The True Cost of the Problem and a Solution

*The statistical information below has been sourced from the Office of National Statistics website. Visit www.ons.gov.uk for further resource and detailed analysis of all data sets involved.

Employee absenteeism is a hot topic and a major concern for the economy. It is for this very reason that companies are seeking ways to minimise and mitigate the issue. One way is through the introduction and implementation of the use of employee benefits packages and the provision of company health insurance schemes and cash plans.

Anything that can be used to assist a company to ensure that the workforce is healthy and well looked after in the event of a medical issue is another tool to be used.

According to the Office for National Statistics, 137.3 million working days were lost due to sickness or injury in the UK in 2016. This is equivalent of 4.3 days per worker.

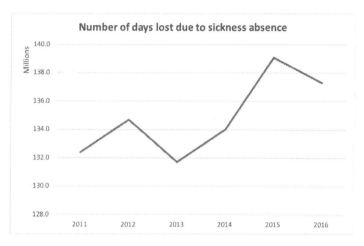

Figure 1. Number of days lost due to sickness absence, UK, 2011-2016. Source: Labour Force Survey – Office for National Statistics

Minor illnesses were the most common reason for absence accounting for approximately 34 million days lost (24.8% of total days lost).

This was followed by musculoskeletal problems (including back pain, neck and upper limb problems) at 30.8 million days (22.4%). After 'other' conditions, mental health issues (including stress, depression, anxiety and serious conditions) were the next most common reason for sickness absence, resulting in 15.8 million days lost (11.5%).

These categories were also the most common reasons given by people for a sickness absence. Minor illnesses were given as a reason for sick absence 33.1% of the time with musculoskeletal problems being reported 18.6% of the time.

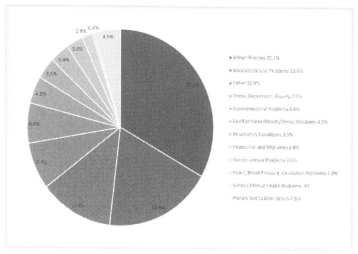

Source: Labour Force Survey – Office for National Statistic

Notes:

'Musculoskeletal problems' includes back pain, neck and upper limb problems and other musculoskeletal problems. 'Other' includes the total number of days lost to diabetes as well as days lost to accidents, poisonings, infectious diseases, skin disorders and anything else not covered. 'Respiratory conditions' include asthma, Chronic Obstructive Pulmonary Disease [OPD], bronchitis and pneumonia. 'Genito-urinary problems' include urine infections, menstrual problems and pregnancy problems.

The groups who experienced the highest rates of sickness absence were women, older workers, those with long-term health conditions, smokers, public health sector workers and those working in the largest organisations (those with 500 or more employees).

Avoiding Employee Absence by Having Private Medical Insurance in Place

As we have already mentioned in previous chapters, having a company private medical insurance in place provides its members fast access to specialists, diagnosis and treatment of medical issues (subject to the insurer and policy benefits) allowing them to return to work quickly and to reduce the lost labour cost to the company.

Interestingly according to The Chartered Institute of Personnel Development (CIPD) Absence Management Survey 2016 found that the average number of lost working days due to sickness per employee, per year, sits at 6.3. Seemingly even higher than the figures from the Office of National Statistics. *CIPD Qualifying statement: There is considerable variation in reported levels of absence, with some organisations reporting very high absence. In order to avoid a few extreme cases skewing the results, we report the 5% trimmed mean.

The same survey found that the absence levels are costing approximately £522 per employee per year in lost working hours (with the survey showing costs to be even higher in the public sector at £835).

If you have 10 employees that's £5,220 annually, with 100 employees the stats show this could cost you up to £52,200 annually, and if you have 1000 employees it's £522,000. That's real money!

These costs are further compounded when you take into account the cost of recruiting new employees as a result or taking on temporary workers.

These statistics and figures are precisely the reason why it is so crucial to put in place suitable programmes and policies to support and maintain the health and wellbeing of the workforce and why it is so crucial that businesses engage with the available solutions on at least some level.

Additionally, on top of the obvious reasons of how a cash plan or health insurance policy would assist an employee to be treated, many plans now offer the addition of wellbeing programmes that promote and allow employees to be more actively involved in healthier lifestyles and also be rewarded for doing so. Some insurers also offer discounts for various gym chains and other services that contribute overall to a healthier workforce, sense of wellbeing and assist them to live healthier lifestyles that may assist in preventing ill health.

The idea that a company should do everything it can to promote wellbeing and good health and do its utmost to prevent absenteeism due to ill health is a no-brainer as it directly affects the profitability of the business.

All this is aside from the fact that the provision of a suitable plan forms part of an overall wellbeing package that promotes loyalty, employee satisfaction and serves as a great tool to attract and retain great talent. Adding further value to your business as it grows and seeks more profitability.

It is clear that health insurance is seen as a very favourable and desired employee benefit to receive and is valued greatly by employees.

CHAPTER 5

How to Select a Broker

The importance of having a health insurance broker you can trust and rely on to evaluate, understand and look after your needs is of utmost importance. This is ever more pertinent when dealing with health insurance which is a complex product that does not lend itself to simplistic comparisons and where a basic level of knowledge just doesn't cut it.

A good broker should be experienced and knowledgeable, have a strong relationship with insurers, account managers and underwriters, be fully compliant, have a highly competent level of knowledge on what the market offers, the various products, nuances surrounding cover and underwriting stances and be fully available to offer advice.

It goes without saying that a good broker should not leave you stranded and be ready to assist you if you need to make a claim or have a claims-related issue.

Care should also be taken when considering cashback offers, 'months free' incentives or special offers from insurers. This may seem attractive initially, however it may not suit your needs long-term and if in doubt a second opinion should always be sought in this instance. Where things check out, by all means, enjoy the extra benefits available.

When engaging a broker, you should look for him or her to use the following best practices:

1. Start with a relaxed, yet thorough conversation to gather the facts, assess your needs, and help you determine how health insurance best supports your goals. It's critical that any broker you engage with listens to your needs, and helps you understand the options available.

2. Complete a fair and personal analysis of the market by comparing products from a wide range of insurers, based on your specific requirements, taking into consideration your business goals, needs and budget.

3. Present findings in a clear and comprehensible way (without using "insurance jargon"), so that you understand all your options, and the advantages and disadvantages of each product and plan. As well as a clear recommendation.

4. Once your application is approved and you are insured, your broker should continue to provide care and support throughout the life of your health insurance policy. Inevitably, questions about coverage, claims processes and assistance, premium payments, and policy terms come up. You want to know that an answer is a quick and easy phone call away (no long delays waiting on hold and talking to someone who cannot answer your questions). You want to know that you have direct access to your broker.

Your broker's job is to act as an intermediary to ensure that you are able to navigate the complexities of finding a suitable policy and to simplify the process through suitable guidance and research.

So, what exactly should you consider during your discussions with an intermediary?

You should ask yourself what your budget is, and how much you can conceivably spend. How comprehensive do you want your cover to be? Do you want to have the choice of treatment in the top tier hospitals, or would you be happy for the employees to have any treatment in a hospital available from a more limited range chosen by your insurance company?

Also, you might want to look at what you are not covered for. Too often people misunderstand the exact terms of cover when taking out a policy, only to find out later they are not covered as expected. The terms and exclusions should be clearly explained by your broker before you agree to taking out the plan.

It is helpful although not mandatory, if your broker has the industry qualifications called the IF7 exam, after all you want to work with an intermediary committed to their own professional development.

Also, although not mandatory, it might be advantageous to use an intermediary who is a member of the AMII. The Association of Medical Insurers and Intermediaries (AMII) was established in 1998 as a trade association for independent medical insurance advisers in the UK. It has more than 120 professional intermediaries advising on health and wellbeing matters, including group risk, and has more than 15 corporate members who are the providers and insurers of Health Cash Plans and Private Medical Insurance.

AMII promotes and maintains high standards of professional and ethical conduct among its members in order to inspire the confidence of the client, no matter whether they be individuals, small and medium-sized enterprises or corporate buyers of health, wellbeing and risk services.

All AMII members are authorised and regulated by either the Prudential Regulatory Authority (PRA) or Financial Conduct Authority (FCA) to sell general insurance products.

If you are seeking independent advice on health insurance products - either for yourself, your family or your business - use the website to Find an Expert or Ask an Expert feature at www.amii.org.uk.

CHAPTER 6

What Should Happen at your Company Health Insurance Renewal?

If you are an existing company health insurance policy-holder, you will know that approximately 6-8 weeks prior to the annual renewal date, the insurer releases the renewal premium for the coming year along with notification of any changes in the policy benefits.

As intermediaries, we receive copies of the renewal invitation documents and we assist with managing the renewal on our clients' behalf. There is a process we follow to endeavour to meet our clients' needs by recommending the product that is most suited to their requirements for the next policy year.

I have detailed the steps below, so you can know exactly what you should expect from a broker. Processes will differ slightly but ultimately things should be covered off as follows:

The Renewal Review

We receive the renewal details, including any premium changes and new policy documents.

We contact the client to carry out a detailed fact find (this happens each year) so we can ensure that any changes to be made are actioned. Multiple changes can occur during the year, so it is important we can keep track and advise accordingly.

We check and confirm with the client the policy member listing to account for group leavers/joiners/retirees, employee promotions, over age dependents, births or, unfortunately at times, divorce or deaths. There may also be historic and on-going claims and medical conditions the group secretary is aware of that can impact our advice. It is important to mention however, that it is not a requirement of the group secretary to ask for employees' private or sensitive information and I am referring to situations where this is knowledge already known to the group secretary.

Also, the company's actual needs may have changed in terms of the kind of employee benefits package they wish to offer the workforce. They may wish to increase or decrease cover, change benefits, excess amounts and hospital listings, the allocated budget may have adjusted, or the client may be unhappy with the incumbent insurer and wish to explore other options in line with their ever-changing needs.

Whatever it is, the fact-finding process is an important discussion that needs to take place so that the renewal review can be carried out in accordance with the situation at hand and achieve the best outcome for the client.

Trusted Advice

With the updated fact find we begin to formulate the basis of our advice. We will have discussions with the incumbent insurer to discuss the risk profile, any changes and apply for discounts where possible.

Where applicable we also complete a market review. This involves a manual process of procuring quotes from each of the relevant insurance providers, collating and having multiple negotiations to ensure the most favorable premiums have been offered by insurers. In my office, we take this very seriously, leaving no stone unturned to achieve the best outcomes. This is a simplified description of what we do and there are many methods, tools and techniques we use to do this.

The review is then collated in a comprehensive, easy to understand report and sent to the client. The report shows the full picture, our review and our final professional recommendation for the coming year. By example, the recommendation may be to remain with the current insurer, make some adjustments, restructure the policy or move to another insurance provider if beneficial for the client.

Explanation of the Market

Importantly, we then follow up to carefully explain what has taken place, answer any questions and guide the client on making a final decision. On the client's agreement to proceed we then process the renewal accordingly, informing the insurers about any changes or adjustments whilst ensuring that that the cover is arranged with minimum fuss.

If there is a switch to another provider, we will also arrange this, ensuring the transfer is smooth, taking care of all paperwork and certificates required to facilitate the switch.

Ongoing Care and Support

We continually follow up, always letting the client know what stage we are up to in the process. We also ensure the correct insurer documentation reaches the client and our Statement of Demands and Needs are sent out in a timely fashion and ensure the client has everything needed for the coming policy year.

Where suitable, we will visit the client and carry out a presentation so that the employees are educated on the benefits of the policy. Employees greatly value this as they truly feel the company is looking after them.

Ultimately it is about protecting the workforce, giving them peace of mind and fostering a strong sense of care, loyalty and workplace happiness. We may also visit with an insurer to assist with the presentation.

What to Avoid

I have seen some awful renewals where no fact find has been completed and the adviser has not taken the time to understand what it is the client actually requires. Cases regularly land on my desk where the broker has done zero work on behalf of the client, expecting it to just renew. These are cases where I have seen no communication with the incumbent insurer, no attempt to lower the cost whatsoever and certainly no market review.

Normally we can extricate the clients from these unhelpful scenarios, show them better options and give them the care and service they ought to be getting from their current intermediary. Clients are normally surprised at what can be done on their behalf when things are addressed properly and accordingly, are most grateful.

If premiums are not managed carefully at the annual renewal and simply allowed to roll over at the increased renewal premium set by the insurer, clients run the risk of having unnecessary premium increases year on year and ultimately, a few years later find themselves being asked to pay exceptionally high premiums. This can be easily avoided if they review their policy annually and where possible maintain the lowest premiums possible. It goes without saying this is in addition to making sure that the cover in place actually suits the requirements of the client effectively.

A broker that does not communicate properly, delays sending the client the review until last minute, or does not complete a review properly or at all, does a huge disservice to the profession and to the client.

CHAPTER 7

How to Make Your Employee Benefits Package Attractive (and why you will want to)

Your benefits package is not just a "gift" to employees, but also a strategic asset you use to attract the talent you need to keep your business growing.

In this chapter I would like to outline some other main elements of what can comprise an employee benefits package. Not all packages will include all the options below, rather one or a few options depending on needs, preference and cost and although this book is centred around the provision of private healthcare, it is important to point out that there are other pieces of the jigsaw to consider.

If you want to have further relevant advice on any of the options below please get in touch with me, isaac@lifepointhealthcare.co.uk and I would be happy to put you in touch with one of my colleagues who specialises in the relevant area.

It is important to point out that there are numerous insurance providers, with variations on products and benefit types, so the below is intended as a very general and broad guide of what the market offers.

Employee Benefits that Offer Protection Against Illness, Accident, Injury or Death

- *Private Medical Insurance (PMI) otherwise known as Health Insurance*

As this book has described, this product goes toward the cost of paying for private medical treatment and allows the policyholder to be seen quickly by specialists, at a location and time of choosing and treated accordingly so that employees can be back at work as soon as possible. It is important to note that the specialists and treatment must be recognised by the insurer and authorised by the insurer before any treatment goes ahead.

- *Critical Illness Insurance*

In the event of an employee being diagnosed with one of certain specific critical illnesses, the employee can receive a tax-free lump sum if they survive for a minimum period of time. Examples of conditions covered are heart issues, cancer and stroke. Insurers will have different definitions, so it is important to be guided on this by an expert. This lump sum can go a long way with helping to assist with costs, whatever they may be. Certainly it can be helpful in assisting with the costs of illness and associated life changes.

- *Group Income Protection (GIP)*

In the event an employee can no longer work due to injury or long-term illness, income protection will pay a percentage of their salary as a regular monthly income. Normally payments begin after a certain period of time off work, however an employer can choose, from the options offered by the insurer, when they want the benefits to kick in.

A variation of this cover can also be a short-term income protection plan called Sick Pay Insurance and this can provide short-term financial support for sickness absence. The waiting period can be shorter (even as little as one week) and works well when set up alongside a company's existing longer-term income protection scheme.

- *Life Insurance – also called Death in Service*

In the event of an employee dying, this product pays a tax-free lump sum to their family and dependants. The amount of benefit is quite often calculated as a multiple of their salary, e.g. if an employee earned £50,000, and the 4 times salary benefit was chosen, the family would receive a £200,000 lump sum. The amount can be used to support the family and acts as a protective financial buffer.

- *Dental and Optical Insurance*

These plans are very popular and go towards paying the cost of routine dental and optical treatment. The dental benefits can range from routine examinations, fillings, polishing and crowns and extend (depending on product and cover levels) to dental injuries and more serious forms of dental treatment. The optical cover can go towards the reimbursement of glasses, contact lenses and eye tests. Some insurers also include these benefits, as an option, within a private medical insurance plan obviating a need for a separate plan alongside it.

- **Health Cash Plans**

A cash plan is a lower cost healthcare plan option that is designed to cover the everyday healthcare costs that you pay directly to the provider of your choice. The cash plan is usually paid for by the company, for the benefit of the members of the scheme. It allows the employee to claim back the cost of treatments, such as optical tests, dental treatment and physiotherapy. You pay a monthly premium, ranging from as little as £5 a month to £65 + per member depending on the options and benefit level chosen. The plan lets the employee claim all or a proportion of the money back.

Company cash plans are extremely affordable and easily accessible.

- **Health Screening**

Health screening allows employees to have health checks and medical examinations and can form part of a pre-emptive approach to healthcare. It allows the employee to be more health aware through the proposal of various lifestyle changes and could also lead to the diagnosis of a medical condition that was undetected, prior to the screening. Appropriate treatment can then commence.

- **Additional Benefits**

In addition to the above, there are other benefits such as workplace pensions, workplace ISAs, share schemes, car allowances, childcare vouchers, gym memberships and employee benefit discount portals that can be offered.

We also have a bespoke discount portal we offer free of charge to our company health insurance clients which offers thousands of pounds of discounts and savings on retail, leisure, health and wellbeing, travel and finance. The company employees find this incredibly useful. All part of the service of providing clients the tools to increase employee happiness.

Solving the Puzzle

All company needs are different, and what works for one may not work for another.

Here's why this is such a complex issue:

Employees in certain industries and company sizes may have expectations about the level of the employee benefits offered and some not so much. These expectations are taken into account by prospective employees when exploring job opportunities and comparing different roles on offer. And the benefits can sometimes make all the difference, so it is important this part of the employee satisfaction process is not relegated to the unimportant.

Ultimately this all comes back to the fact-finding process and allowing a specialist to truly assess the needs of the firm so that they can be met, or at least explored accordingly.

Employee benefits are indeed like assembling a large jigsaw puzzle. Misplace one piece and you cannot complete the picture. I urge you to get help from a competent professional— from our firm, or another...just get the help you need.

CHAPTER 8

What to do Next

If you are approaching your health insurance renewal, contact me and my team at Lifepoint Healthcare. A "second opinion" can never hurt. Our goal is to ensure you have the right health insurance plan, that delivers all of the benefits you want for your employees and does so at the right price. Our 4 Step process (Chapter 6) will give you greater clarity around the cover you really need, and your options for custom-tailoring a plan to your specific needs and desires. *If you are ready to add health insurance* to your employee benefits offering, the best place to start is with a brief meeting by phone or in person. At this stage, it's critical that you get clear on the type of cover that is most important to you, so that a plan can be customised for your company.

In either case, the best next step is to schedule a brief appointment.
Schedule by phone: 020 33489868
Schedule by email: isaac@lifepointhealthcare.co.uk
My team and I look forward to speaking with you.

TESTIMONIALS

Dear Isaac, we wish to take this opportunity to thank you for arranging the additional cover of Dental and Optical on top of our Private Healthcare which you organise. We also appreciate your excellent service addressed to every member of our staff.

With best regards,
Holly Chong
Shanghai Commercial Bank

Lifepoint Healthcare continues to look after our firm's private healthcare & employee benefits. They always have our best interests in mind, consistently take the time to ensure we have the most suitable cover in place (at the best value) for our staff & are always on hand to assist us where necessary during the year as well, be it claims, guidance or other.

It is a pleasure knowing we are in safe hands and are grateful to Isaac & his exceptional team.

David Finn, Partner
RDP Newmans

Dear Isaac, I am just dropping you a short note to express my sincere thanks and deep appreciation for all your efforts in arranging healthcare for me in view of the difficulties I had just experienced. Not only were you able to achieve a very competitive premium from a reputable insurer but your prompt attention (always returning my calls) and genuine helpfulness and input were added bonuses. In short, it was a pleasure dealing with you and I would have no hesitation to highly recommending you to other potential clients.

J Gutstein
FPCS Stonelink Investment Management Ltd

Lifepoint is a great health insurance intermediary. When I joined a few months ago, Isaac spent time in obtaining and then negotiating quotes with the insurance companies. His personal and expert service ensured we achieved the right level of cover and the best price for us. We would unreservedly recommend his services.

Dr. Simon Freilich
Consultant in Clinical Neurophysiology
at the Hospital of St John & St Elizabeth

Isaac has provided an outstanding quote for a 'fully loaded' policy that beat all competitors, and his service does not end there... His aftercare service is truly heartwarming.

Jeremy Lloyd
Western Circle Ltd

After searching for a healthcare intermediary, we are thrilled to have found Isaac Feiner at Lifepoint Healthcare.

Isaac spent as much time as was needed explaining all our options in depth and endeavoured to find us the best product for our young family. Whenever we have had any queries, he has always been on hand to help and advise with haste and care.

An outstanding firm with its customers at its core, a firm that I have recommended to lots of friends and family.

Dalia Nessim
Physio Clinic London – The Wellington

Excellent pricing, speedy response, transparent advice & impartial quotations. Well done. A satisfied client.

Norman Feiner
Simply Fone Ltd

I am very happy to recommend Isaac Feiner of Lifepoint Healthcare. He is very knowledgeable and offers a highly professional service. He shows great care and concern for his clients and is a pleasure to deal with.

Rev Michael Binstock, MBE Director
Jewish Prison Chaplaincy

Lifepoint Healthcare undertook a free review of our Private Medical policy and found we could save a huge amount of money and have better protection at the same time!

We switched to Lifepoint and haven't looked back. Apart from the savings and the great cover, the customer service element is second to none. Assisting with specific claims and expediting authorisations has added to the great value Lifepoint has given to First Union. First Union promotes great services and we expect that from our partners – Lifepoint Healthcare has lived up to that expectation.

Meir Plancey, Director
First Union Mortgages

We have worked with Lifepoint for over a year now and have always found them very efficient, informative and friendly. Am always shocked at the speed they come back to me with a quote and answering any queries we may have. I would 100% recommend them to any colleagues requesting their services.

Mel
Percy & Reed Salons – Great Portland Street

Lifepoint Healthcare is an appointed representative of Premier Choice Healthcare Ltd which is authorised and regulated by the Financial Conduct Authority.

FCA ref: 662989 and 312878.